Gino Lemos
Charles Martins

BIOMECHANICS IN HORSES

Gino Lemos
Charles Martins

BIOMECHANICS IN HORSES

Literature review on the kinesiological aspects of
athletic horses

ScienciaScripts

BIOMECHANICS IN HORSES

Literature review on the kinesiological aspects of athletic horses

Gino Luigi Bonilla Lemos Pizzi

Charles Ferreira Martins

ABOUT THE AUTHORS

Charles Ferreira Martins - He has a degree and a master's degree in Veterinary Medicine from the Federal University of Pelotas (UFPel) and a doctorate from the São Paulo State University Júlio de Mesquita Filho. He is currently a professor in the Veterinary Clinic Department and a permanent member of the Postgraduate Program in Zootechnics at the Federal University of Pelotas (UFPel) in the area of equine biomechanics, as well as Director of the Veterinary Clinic Hospital at the Federal University of Pelotas and Coordinator of the Equine Orthopedics Study Group.

E-mail: martinscf68@yahoo.com.br

Gino Luigi Bonilla Lemos Pizzi - Graduated in Veterinary Medicine from the Federal University of Pelotas - UFPel, Master's degree from the Federal University of Pelotas - UFPel in the Postgraduate Program in Animal Science, in the area of Animal Production (CNPq scholarship). PhD in Animal Production from the Postgraduate Program in Zootechnics/UFPel, with a focus on equine biomechanics and kinematics, with a Sandwich PhD period (CAPES - Print) at the School of Veterinary Physiotherapy at Writtle University College, in the United Kingdom, from 2022 to 2023.

E-mail: gino_lemos@hotmail.com

SUMMARY

This book offers a comprehensive overview of equine biomechanics and physiology, covering everything from the basics of anatomy and locomotion to more specific issues related to athletic performance and injury prevention. Initially, the fundamental principles of equine biomechanics are explored, highlighting the importance of understanding the kinematics and kinetics of movements in athletic horses. This includes detailed analysis of gaits and specific movements during riding, providing a solid basis for understanding the biomechanical aspects related to sports performance.

The book then looks at the functional anatomy of equine limbs, examining in detail the structure and function of bones, joints and muscles. It highlights the importance of the specific biomechanics of the different joints and muscle groups in the context of equine locomotion, offering valuable insights for trainers, veterinarians and professionals in the field. It also explores the anatomy and biomechanics of the axial skeleton, with a focus on the equine neck, trunk and spine. It discusses the function of the muscles involved in supporting the trunk between the thoracic limbs, as well as the importance of spinal mobility for athletic performance and injury prevention.

All in all, this book provides an in-depth understanding of the biomechanical and physiological aspects that influence the performance and well-being of horses, and is an enjoyable and essential read for all those involved in the care and training of these animals.

Keywords: kinesiology, musculoskeletal system, kinematics, kinetics.

CHAPTER 1

EVOLUTION OF STUDIES IN EQUINE BIOMECHANICS

The field of studies on the ability of living beings to move to meet their physiological needs is extremely broad and complex. In veterinary medicine, it can be said that it began with the first specific vocational colleges, in the Lyon and Paris region of France, in the mid-1761s and 1765s. Van Weeren (2012) described that the initial studies were artistic and were based on paintings depicting equine animals in slower, more moderate movements, as well as diagrammatic drawings of limbs to help students study. The author also discussed the difficulties encountered in evaluating faster gaits (*e.g.* galloping), due to the difficulty of the human eye in capturing images in very short time intervals, such as the rapid change of position of the limbs.

Within this context, the evolution of observational studies of equine gait came with the advent of photography and Eadweard Muybridge's experiment, which revolutionized both the direction of image capture and the understanding that horses go through a phase of flight in the canter, consisting of no support on the ground, due to the powerful propulsion of the body at high speeds (Muybridge, 1957; Ott, 2005; Egan *et al.*, 2019). Until the Second World War, which brought important updates with the use of electronic equipment for the study of equine movement, it was considered the first great era of gait analysis in the species, and the animals of this species experienced a drop in their numbers due to their intense use in battles over the decades. It was only in the post-war period that the horse began to be seen as a leisure and sport animal, completely changing the status that the different breeds and categories occupied with anthropic activities, giving rise to the second great era of movement analysis (Slijper, 1946; Van Weeren *et al.*, 2000).

The advent of computerized technologies has expanded the field of biomechanical research in animals (Mchenry & Hendrick, 2023), including the equine species. The ability to obtain images that allow the analysis of rapid movements that are intangible to the human eye has facilitated more detailed and objective observation of the different moments of the stride in the most diverse categories of athletic horses (Van Weeren, 2012). For Egan *et al.* (2019), research trends in recent decades suggest that knowledge creation is driven by technology, due to the fact that in the early 1990s, much of the published research into equine gait analysis focused on the development of studies based on 2D video, optical motion capture systems and force platforms. This continued until around the end of that decade, when wearable sensors began to be developed, positioned directly on the animal in widespread research practice, validating the use of these technologies, as it was a more practical and applicable way of doing things in the field.

In 1973, with the establishment of the *International Society of Biomechanics (ISB)*, the term biomechanics was defined as "the examination of the structures and functions of biological systems using mechanical approaches" (Hatze, 1974). This field of study aims to analyze the loads, movements, stresses and deformations in biological systems, which can include humans, animals, plants or combinations thereof, as well as the mechanical effects on the movement, size, shape and structure of these systems (Lu & Chang, 2012). Biomechanics is an interdisciplinary field that integrates the principles of mechanics, biology and physiology.

Currently, research into applied equine biomechanics is a growing trend due to the high variability of breeds and categories of athletic animals, which has led to an exponential growth in literature on the subject in recent decades (Barrey, 1999;

Von Peinen *et al.*, 2009). Depending on the focus of each research group, studies can differentiate between those aimed at determining the load subjected to the biomechanics of internal structures of the equine musculoskeletal system, with the main objective of preventing and reducing injuries, and also investigations examining the horse-rider interaction, addressing human-induced effects on equestrian activities, as well as those evaluating the effects of any other type of intervention on equine athletes (*e.g.* orthopedic horseshoes) (Dakin *et al.*, 2011; Van Weeren, 2012).

Nevertheless, studies have spread to the most diverse equine categories and breeds around the globe due to the intersection of the use of these individuals in equestrian disciplines, accompanying social development over the years (Adelman & Thompson, 2017). From regional competitions, restricted mainly by the racial factor, to the Olympic Games, the athletic demands of individuals increase with each passing year, extracting the best performance in terms of morphology, speed, strength and endurance; all these characters being worked on in unison and giving the beauty of the equine gait, appreciated worldwide and described since the times of Ancient Greece (Patay-Horváth, 2020). For these reasons, the field of studies on the English Thoroughbred and Quarter Horse breeds has intensified, not only by typifying the biomechanical characteristics of the different gaits performed by these animals, but also in a way that is applicable in the medical clinic to promote methods of prevention and detection of lameness (Leach & Dagg, 1983). In Brazil, the Crioula and Mangalarga Marchadora breeds exemplify categories with their own associations of breeders and competitions at a high level of morphofunctional performance. However, they also illustrate how the level of specific biomechanical research between the two contrasts. In the Mangalarga Marchador breed, there are several studies addressing everything from predicting foal performance in the first few years of life (Soares, 2017; Santos, 2018), to descriptive analysis of the gait of these individuals (Hussni *et al.*, 1996; Fonseca, 2018; Simonato *et al.,* 2021) and including the application of therapeutic methods in horses with orthopedic ailments (Antonioli, 2019; Paz *et al.,* 2019). However, there are still few applications of kinetic and kinematic methods for morphofunctional assessments in Criollo horses.

Van Weeren (2012) goes on to say that capturing the very high frequency and amplitude vibrations that occur distally in the equine appendicular skeleton during ground touch in fast gaits is still very technically demanding. However, the challenge of the last few decades in fundamental equine biomechanics, according to the author, lies not in a better description of what happens, but in discovering the mechanisms and concepts of equine locomotion. The first methodologies established for analyzing equine gait were, for the most part, adapted from what was also used in humans, a fact that still recurs with the new computerized technologies. In 1874, Marey used a system of wired sensors applied to the thoracic and pelvic limbs of horses, which emitted a graphic signal when they touched the ground (Vilela Jr, 2009). In the 1990s, Smith (1996) pioneered the kinematic assessment of equine gait transitions. Barrey (1999) used markers at specific anatomical points to help analyze not only equine biomechanics, but also descriptive measurements of the training track. Advances in computerized techniques have meant that different types of markers can be applied to animals according to need, including the production of virtual markers by *software* specialized in gait analysis (Clayton & Schamhardt, 2001; Bretas *et al.*, 2003). The key point of the new technologies is to associate non-invasive techniques with the animal, with the determination of the biomechanical effects of specific locomotor actions on potentially vulnerable structures of the equine limbs and spine. Egan *et al.* (2019) argue that usually the subjective clinical indicators of lameness are clear bilateral discrepancies between the left and right sides; however, much evidence states that this is only obvious when the initial lameness is severe. A potential solution could be that, according to the authors, instead of simply quantifying gait parameters such as stride times and comparing right and left side movement, the quality of the movement signal can also be examined over time, making the assessment of clinical cases more dynamic, providing *feedback* on the evolution of the case and the treatment applied.

CHAPTER 2

KINEMATIC ANALYSIS IN HORSES

The study of the movement of the locomotor system of living beings is undergoing a considerable revolution with the arrival of new video analysis technologies. Not only do clinical studies begin to be made possible, but diagnoses are also defined with the aid of video, as well as the quantification of different treatments for different injuries and illnesses. Torres-Pérez *et al.* (2016) point out that, despite the exponential growth of these dynamic measurement technologies since the 1990s, there are still not many systems designed specifically for the equine species, since they are derived from *software* and *hardware* applied to humans, making it difficult for many clinical centers around the world, which care for a large number of sick animals, to make quantitative assessments to typify the gaits of different diseases and evaluate the progression of treatments.

In kinemetry, to investigate the position and orientation of body segments, there are two types of systems for capturing and analyzing videos, in relation to the coverage of more spatial dimensions in the field of filming, these being 2D and 3D. The two-dimensional system captures gait in the sagittal plane, using just one camera and a more simplified measurement and data processing system, ideal for specific diseases in clinical routine, as it requires less time to set up and apply (Castelli *et al.*, 2015). According to Clayton & Schamhardt (2001), in two-dimensional studies angular data is generally reported as flexion and extension in the sagittal plane. This could be a reasonable simplification of why the horse's joints have evolved to move mainly in this plane, as an energy-saving mechanism. The three-dimensional system, on the other hand, represents a much more precise and sensitive analysis of movement in all three planes, requiring the use of multi-cameras positioned at 360° to fully gauge the gaits performed by the individuals, requiring more time for set-up and calibration before application and thus making it a more costly method (Baker, 2006; Ceseracciu *et al.*, 2014; Sandau *et al.*, 2014).

Michelini *et al.* (2020) also argue that one of the key points when comparing 2D and 3D biomechanical analysis technologies is the need for trained personnel, both in positioning markers at anatomical points of interest and in setting up and calibrating the study field. For the authors, a study with greater sensitivity and validation is the result of adequate training to reduce the margins of interpretation error in the variability of the data collected. In this context, the two-dimensional system becomes simpler and more reliable for operators with a good knowledge of the anatomy of the musculoskeletal system, as it is essential to choose the correct points to be assessed using video. The reliability of the kinematic analysis also depends on the correct choice of markers. Most 2D systems have a diameter of around 1 to 3 cm and are photosensitive, i.e. their image is captured by the camera when natural or artificial light is shone on it, with a spherical shape that allows the central point to be determined, referring to the anatomical point on which it was positioned (Chung & Ng, 2012). Three-dimensional systems basically work by emitting infrared light from the camera system to the markers, which have specific material to reflect it back.

Although the reliability of the 3D method is greater, due to the details already mentioned, the high cost, the time required for assembly and calibration and the need for an accurately trained team to validate the data collected, makes it difficult to apply this methodology in the clinical routine, not only for the reality of equine sports veterinary medicine, but also in medicine (Ugbolue *et al.*, 2013; Castelli *et al.*, 2015). As such, the 2D system, a precursor of kinematic analysis since the last century with the advent of photography and, later, video taking, continues to have a place and is a viable and reliable alternative for clinical investigations of bilateral changes in different gaits, as well as the rehabilitation of injuries with ongoing treatment (Whittle, 1996; Baker, 2006). The main data collected with this method are the linear and angular spatiotemporal displacements, i.e. the change in movement in the sagittal plane that the anatomical markers promote in a pre-defined stride cycle in the software calibration (De Godoi *et al.*, 2014). This specific movement basically refers to the vertical and horizontal displacement (m/s) in relation to the total time of the analyzed stride, as well as the changes in angulation (°/s) that a synovial joint promotes in the different phases of the stride. However, important information such as stride length (m) and gait time (s) is also captured and processed by motion analysis systems. This data is usually captured bilaterally, i.e. by positioning the anatomical markers at equal points on the right and left sides, in order to detect biomechanical inconsistencies when comparing both sides. This form of motion capture requires at least one camera, with the animal passing through both lateral views, with the alternative of filming bilaterally, positioning a second camera with the same calibration on the contralateral side. There is also the possibility of the operator correcting and adding virtual markers during the analysis via *software* to mitigate possible collection defects caused by markers falling off due to sweat or poor attachment to the animal's fur.

The types of cameras that can be used in two-dimensional systems vary according to the evolution of technology. In recent decades, high-motion capture (RGB) cameras have given way to *smartphones* with equal or superior filming capacity at frequencies of up to 120Hz, making this methodology portable and applicable to the field, expanding the range of animals that can have their gaits analyzed, without the need for a specific physical laboratory to collect biomechanical data.

The applicability of the kinematic study in equine athletes has the most varied nuances of investigation, from the typification of gait in certain categories of animals, through bilateral analysis to detect biomechanical incongruities that alter performance, characterization of gait in specific locomotor diseases and the influence of different saddle positions and the rider himself working the horse (Meershoek *et al.*, 2001; Martin *et al.,* 2016; Egan *et al.,* 2019; Dyson et *al.,* 2020).

Pfau (2019) argues that the use of cameras can quantify movement, both in the upper body and in the more distal portions, even though there are methodological challenges to implementing this system, due to the nature, in particular, of distal limb movements involving high accelerations during impact of the hoof surface, stationary periods during support and high rotational speeds during movement. The author also mentions that the comparatively large margins of error shown in published validation studies (Olsen *et al.*, 2013; Roepstorff *et al.,* 2013) and repeatability coefficients of several degrees (Cruz *et al.*, 2017) reinforce the challenge, not only of using kinemetrics, but also inertial sensors for validating accelerometer analysis. With camera-based limb movement measurements, it will finally be possible to investigate which parameters have the best sensitivity and specificity for detecting specific types of lameness, i.e. it will be possible to determine whether specific injuries are related to changes in gait patterns, and the typification of certain diseases in animals of different categories is becoming a trend in research around the world.

CHAPTER 3

KINETIC ANALYSIS IN HORSES

Movement is an important indicator of an individual's functional capacity and general health, and reflects the integrity of the physiological systems as a whole, making it of fundamental importance to analyze it in order to assess the impacts of health conditions (Allum & Adkin, 2003; Alsiri *et al.*, 2020). Since locomotion is an action through interaction with the environment, there are forces exerted to initiate, maintain or alter movement that produce a reaction, based on physical laws that form the basis of classical mechanics (Clayton & Hobbs, 2019). During riding movements, the magnitude and direction of the forces exerted by the horse, through contact with the hoof and ground, are balanced by an equal force acting in the opposite direction. During locomotion, therefore, as the hooves press on the ground during the support phase, the ground pushes back on the hooves with a force of equal magnitude acting in the opposite direction, respecting Newton's third law, and this is called the *ground reaction forces* (GRF) (Gustås *et al.*, 2004). In this context, there are specific methods for quantifying and measuring the interaction of these forces and their impact on the musculoskeletal system of equine individuals.

The main technique for measuring the kinetic forces acting on the gait of living beings is dynamometry, which is the objective assessment of the functional force and impact exerted on a body segment, where the deforming action is measured using a direct method that determines the external forces, which are necessary prerequisites for calculating the internal forces (muscle, ligament and joint forces) (Hill *et al.*, 2005; Munoz-Nates *et al.*, 2015). The result of the conditions of the training and competition tracks of equine athletes also translates into musculoskeletal injuries, causing disability in these individuals (Henley *et al.*, 2006). Therefore, quantifying the effect of GRF on the locomotor system of these categories is of paramount importance in order to assess risk factors for animal welfare, reducing the incidence of injuries and improving athletic performance.

For many decades, force and pressure platforms have been used, as they measure a wide range of effects on the horse, such as the disproportionate distribution of x, y and z forces, as well as changes in posture and balance, with the ability to record forces of more than a ton in the animal's gallop, making them a valuable clinical tool (Pratt & O'connor, 1976). However, these devices were restricted to research centers due to their inability to be portable. Then, the new wearable technologies of horseshoes and rugs with piezoelectric sensors allowed for the recording of numerical and graphical data that was previously difficult, or even impossible, to obtain with conventional force platforms; this ended up providing important information for evaluating the biomechanical consequences and risk factors associated with the properties of the track surface in racehorses, as well as the application and positioning of the saddle and rider and even the effects of bridle pressure and embouchure on the performance of the equine athlete (Chateau *et al., 2009; Robin et al.,* 2009), 2009; Robin *et al.,* 2009; Murray *et al.,* 2015; Martin et *al.,* 2016; Nocera *et al.,* 2021).

In a more experimental way, anthropometry provides non-invasive methods for quantitative measurements of the human body, and it is a model that has had several applications in horses over the years (Casadei & Kiel, 2020). Liley *et al.* (2017) argue that medical imaging modalities, such as computed tomography and magnetic resonance imaging, are expensive and difficult to perform on live animals, and are often inaccessible in many medical centers. Within this scenario, anthropometry determines the characteristics and properties of the locomotor system, such as the geometric shape of body segments, mass distribution, lever arms and joint positions, through models so that the forces of origin can be inferred (inverse dynamics) and the center of mass can be estimated (Amadio & Duarte, 1996; Graziano, 2008). However, according to Scafoglieri *et al.* (2014), there are limitations to the use of this technique for the applicability of these data in clinical practice, such as measurement error by the evaluators, as well as inter- and intra-observer variability, ranging from 3% to 24% of the results obtained. Other authors have also argued that there are more up-to-date techniques for obtaining quantitative results from body measurements applied directly to individuals, as well as individual factors that directly interfere with the extrapolation of data obtained directly from a reference model, such as age, weight, gender, physical activity, among others (Ulijaszek & Kerr, 1999; Park *et al.*, 2009). In addition, unlike humans, it is very challenging to keep a horse still, and the distinct anatomy of these individuals denotes traits that cannot be measured on the surface (e.g. shoulder joint, at the most caudal point of the scapula), since they lie under layers of adipose tissue and muscle in the bones of a horse (Thomas *et al.*, 2014). All these positive and negative factors should be considered and debated when choosing the correct modeling for anthropometric investigations in horses.

Finally, electromyography (EMG), according to Mills (2005), consists of recording the electrical activity of the muscle, with the ability to distinguish myopathic from neurogenic muscle loss and weakness. According to the author, the test can detect abnormalities such as chronic denervation or fasciculations in clinically normal muscles, as well as differentiating focal nerve, plexus or root pathology. The signal captured by EMG is the electrical manifestation of neuromuscular activation, associated with a muscle in contraction, which represents the current generated by the ionic flow through the membrane of the muscle fibers, which propagates through the intervening tissues to reach the detection surface of an electrode located in the environment (De Luca, 2006). It is a complicated signal, as it is affected by the anatomical and physiological properties of the muscles and the control scheme of the nervous system, as well as the characteristics of the instrumentation used to detect and observe it.

Basically, there are two types of electromyographic measurement of the muscles of interest, which can consist of either the application of surface electrodes to the skin, which are normally used to assess large and superficial muscles, or wire or needle electrodes, which are used to detect the activity of small and deep muscles, the latter being more suitable for a more reliable assessment of muscle activity, as they are inserted directly into the contractile unit (Sherburn & Bø, 2005; Hug, 2011). However, the use of EMG sensors in horses has its limitations. When superficial electrodes are used, they are limited to the superficial musculature of an individual, and there may be interference in the signal due to displacement of the skin, associated with poor fixation of the electrode, and there is also variation caused by the depth of the subcutaneous adipose tissue, which acts as a filter between the muscle and the sensor, thus reducing the reliability of the source of the detected signal (De Luca *et al.*, 2010; Williams, 2018). Although deep needle EMG systems offer greater specificity and analyze the deep compartment of the muscles, which allows defined areas to be evaluated, they are more invasive systems, since fine wire electrodes are inserted via a hypodermic needle, causing associated discomfort (Kamen & Gabriel, 2009). In addition, potential spasticity can occur in target muscles, altering the data of the signals captured, and the electrodes can break and become trapped in the muscle, restricting and limiting the use of this technique to the laboratory (Rash & Quesada, 2003; Daube & Rubin, 2009). Wijnberg & Franssen (2016) argue that the choice and use of the EMG technique has been constantly applied to a growing number of indications, but only by a small number of equine clinicians, as the collection and interpretation of this data requires a thorough understanding of the physiology and pathogenesis of the muscle unit, and successful application depends on controlling a variety of technical factors and mastering data collection skills. For the authors, the technique allows equine clinicians to draw conclusions about the type and severity of muscular ailments, as well as indicating the likely anatomical location of a lesion and the evolution of the clinical condition.

CHAPTER 4

EQUINE BIOMECHANICS: TYPES OF GAIT

Pereira (2019) describes that the term gait was defined by Uspenskii (1953) as "a complex, rhythmic, automatic and extremely coordinated movement of the limbs and the entire body of the animal, resulting in the production of movement". Clayton (2016) further characterizes a gait as a pattern of coordination between the limbs in a repeated manner, in which each repetition is a stride.

In horses, the terms "symmetrical" and "asymmetrical" are used to describe different types of gaits based on coordination, sequence of events and the movement patterns of the limbs. These terms are commonly used to differentiate between the horse's natural gait and the way it moves (Robilliard *et al.*, 2007).

Symmetrical gaits are those in which the horse mobilizes each limb in a regular and uniformly coordinated pattern (Miró *et al.*, 2006). The two main symmetrical gaits are the stride, a four-stroke movement, which means that each hoof hits the ground independently, where the animal moves its limbs in the sequence of left pelvic, left thoracic, right pelvic and right thoracic, with a moment of suspension between each stride, the natural gait being slower; and the trot, a two-stroke gait, where diagonal pairs of limbs move together. The left thoracic and right pelvic segments move forward simultaneously, followed by the contralateral ones. The trot is faster than the walk and is a common gait used in many equestrian disciplines, as well as being the most effective movement in terms of energy expenditure, since it reuses the elastic energy resulting from tendon mobilization to effect caloric savings (Griffin *et al.*, 2004).

On the other hand, asymmetrical gaits are those in which the individual's limbs do not move in a regular and uniformly coordinated pattern (Hildebrand, 1977). There are two primary asymmetrical gaits: the canter, which has three tempos in which the horse moves the limbs in the sequence of the left pelvic, followed by both thoracic together and then the leading pelvic. The canter is faster than the trot and is commonly used in various riding disciplines; and finally, the gallop, a four-stroke gait, but unlike the walk, it is not uniformly coordinated. It involves a moment of suspension, followed by the leading thoracic limb, the leading pelvic limb, the contralateral pelvic limb and finally the contralateral thoracic limb. The canter is the fastest movement a horse can achieve naturally and is often seen during races, or when horses need to escape quickly. These terms are more widespread in the English language (*gallop* and *canter*), where they better translate the different asymmetrical gaits in horses. In England, during the Middle Ages, pilgrims were seen heading towards Canterbury Cathedral with their horses galloping in a three-stroke pattern. Hence the origin of the term canter. In Portuguese, the term galope is commonly used to abbreviate the asymmetrical and fast gaits performed by equines.

It is important to note that not all horses have the ability to perform all gaits. For example, some equine breeds have intermediate patterns, such as the gait, *piaffe*, *passage* and *tölt* (Back *et al.*, 1995; Clayton *et al.*, 2007). In addition, individuals can have asymmetries in their movements due to injuries or conformational problems, which can affect their movement pattern and performance.

CHAPTER 5

EQUINE BIOMECHANICS: STRIDE PHASES

Equine movement is characterized by the repetition of a movement pattern, which represents a stride divided into a support phase and a suspension or elevation phase. In the first, the limb is characterized by retraction while supported on the ground and in the elevation phase the limb suspends itself, undergoing protraction and preparing for the start of the next step which is when this cycle restarts (Clayton, 2017). The support and suspension phases can be further divided into three subparts each. The cranial part of the support is where the limb is received on the ground, this being the moment of greatest load absorption, occurring after the hoof touches the surface. The load is created by the impact of the individual's weight and the reaction force of the ground. In the intermediate phase of support, the limb is aligned with the vertical and this is when the limb bears the greatest load from the animal's body weight. Subsequently, the segment retracts caudally, preparing for the propulsion of the trunk forward, this being the caudal phase of support. During lifting, the limb protrudes and also passes through three parts, but in a caudocranial direction, with all the joints flexing slightly in the caudal phase. The limb is removed from the ground in the caudal position during retraction. This moment when the hoof is removed from contact with the ground is called the *breakover,* and the faster it occurs, the more accurate the movement for equines. The maximum flexion of the limb will occur in the intermediate phase of the suspension, allowing it to pass forward and, in the cranial phase, the limb extends cranially, protracting to touch the ground, thus completing another full stride and preparing to start a new cycle.

CHAPTER 6

TYPES OF MUSCLE CONTRACTION

The muscular action during each phase of the step means that each one has defined characteristics according to the muscle groups acting with the greatest force. In terms of muscle physiology, the terminology of the type of contraction performed by the muscles has been defined since the 1920s and 1930s, when the three main types of muscle activation were typified: concentric, eccentric (isotonic) and isometric (Faulkner, 2003). Padulo *et al.* (2013) describe isotonic contractions: concentric contraction occurs when the muscle shortens while generating tension. This means that the force produced by the muscle is greater than the external resistance applied to it, resulting in a movement towards contraction; eccentric contraction, on the other hand, is characterized by the muscle tensing while the fibres are unclenched. In this case, the external resistance force is greater than the force produced by the muscle, resulting in control of the movement towards elongation. Isometric contraction, unlike the above, occurs when the muscle generates tension, but there is no change in the length of the muscle or movement resulting from the contraction. In this type of contraction, the force produced by the muscle is equal to the external resistance applied, maintaining a fixed position (Goubel, 1978).

CHAPTER 7

MOVEMENT LEVERS

Ramachandran & Lee (2018) describe the musculoskeletal system as a set of connected levers that allow the body to move. The difference between these is where the force is applied, since they are basically made up of three components: a fulcrum (*e.g.* the joint), this being the pivot point of support that allows movement, the muscular force performed and the resistance of the weight to be overcome.

A first-class lever, also called an interfix lever, is a type of lever where the fulcrum is located between the effort and the load. In the context of the animal body, the fulcrum is often represented by a joint such as the elbow, where the effort is the muscular force applied and the load is the resistance that needs to be overcome. The biomechanical advantage is greater strength and range of movement.

In a second-class (inter-resistant) lever, the load is situated between the fulcrum and the effort. In animals, this means that the joint acts as the fulcrum, the muscular force is the effort and the weight or resistance being moved is between the joint and the muscle applying the force. An example of this is the movement carried out by the common calcaneal tendon in the tarsal region, generating more force but less range of movement.

Finally, the third class lever (interpotent) is where the force is between the fulcrum axis and the resistance to be mobilized. The speed and range of movement are greater in this configuration, but it requires more muscle strength to mobilize. The contraction of the biceps brachii is a classic example of this lever in mammals.

CHAPTER 8

ANATOMY AND BIOMECHANICS OF THE APPENDICULAR SKELETON: THORACIC LIMBS

In order to understand the horse's gait, it is necessary to analyze the mechanics of movement, which, because it is a living being, is called biomechanics (Clayton, 2017). The equine thoracic limbs support, on average, between 57 and 60% of the animal's body weight and are of fundamental importance in absorbing mechanical shocks when in contact with the ground during gait (Hobbs & Clayton, 2013). The center of mass of the thoracic limb is located proximally in the region of the shoulder girdle, next to the muscles that generate the forces to move this segment. The forces generated by these muscle groups are dissipated through tendon extensions, which originate from the muscles and insert into the distal part of the limb, helping to generate movement (Kilbourne & Hoffman, 2013). Among these muscles, we highlight the so-called 'extrinsic muscles', which originate in the thorax or neck and are inserted into the thoracic limb. They promote the union of the thoracic segments to the axis of the body, giving this connection the name sinsarcosis (Payne *et al.*, 2005). In addition, these muscles are of fundamental importance in the protraction and retraction of the appendicular segments (Chateau *et al.*, 2013). These angular movements refer to the actions of limb extension and flexion in relation to the body or to a reference position, usually vertical; commonly, the angles of limb protraction and retraction are defined by the angle formed by the limb axis in relation to the vertical during the stride, the limb axis being defined for the entire limb from the segment formed by the hoof and the scapula (Sapone *et al.*, 2021).

The muscles of the thoracic limb work in different ways at different moments of the gait, and this causes the limbs to extend and flex during the stride. In support, the limb is extended cranially during the cranial phase, the supraspinatus muscles and the long head of the triceps brachii perform eccentric contraction, preventing collapse and exacerbated movements of the shoulder and elbow joints during limb extension. In the intermediate phase, the muscles remain in eccentric contraction, providing stability to the limb to support the weight of the horse, with the flexor muscles of the forearm being extremely important for actively supporting the load submitted by the body weight, transferred through the tendons and ligaments located in the digital portion of the limb (Chateau *et al.*, 2013). During the support phase, the extrinsic latissimus dorsi and ascending pectoralis muscles, which have their insertions on the humerus, contract concentrically, retracting the limb (Payne *et al.*, 2005). These muscles are also responsible for propelling the limb in the caudal phase of support, using the energy generated and stored in the limb's muscles and tendons. At the same time as propulsion, the limb extends and the supraspinatus and triceps brachii muscles contract, widening the joint angles of the shoulder and elbow joints. In order for the distal part of the limb to also extend, the flexor muscles of the forearm perform concentric contraction so that the limb is suspended and extended caudally after the *breakover*. In the suspension phase, the limb begins in a caudally retracted position and is not in contact with the ground, undergoing protraction and preparing for the next stride cycle which will begin as soon as the limb is once again supported on the ground in cranial reception. During this stage, the distal end of the scapula moves cranially by concentric contraction of the brachiocephalic, omotransverse and descending pectoral muscles, while the thoracic trapezius muscle pulls the proximal part of the scapula caudally (Payne *et al.*, 2005). In the caudal phase of the swing, the joint angles of the thoracic limb decrease and the limb moves cranially; the deltoid, brachial and biceps brachii muscles flex the shoulder and elbow joints while the caudal antebrachial muscles flex the distal joints of the limb and the carpus. In the middle phase, joint closure of the limb reaches its maximum peak, flexion of the distal joints of the limb is facilitated by the fact that the limb is in suspension and there are no reaction forces opposing the movement, and then the limb begins to extend cranially in preparation for the next phase of the step. The suspended and cranially protracted limb characterizes the last phase of the stride, which is the cranial phase of the suspension. The concentric contraction of the triceps brachii muscle modulates the movement and enhances the action of the supraspinatus muscle, which synergistically extends the shoulder and elbow joints. Contraction of the forearm extensor muscle group extends the distal part of the limb cranially, causing full extension of the limb (Chateau *et al.*, 2013). In the thoracic limb, the scapula acts as a pendulum during the horse's gait, and its craniocaudal displacement determines the amplitude of the stride, which tends to be greater as the horse's speed of movement increases (Johnson & Moore-Colyer, 2009).

The thoracic limb also has support and stability during the station without the need for direct muscle activation, allowing the animal to distribute forces along the segment without releasing energy. This is known as the passive apparatus. The tendon of origin of the biceps brachii muscle, when passing through the humeral intertuberal grooves, promotes tensioning of the scapulohumeral joint, preventing its angle from closing, with the help of the long head of the triceps brachii, which promotes an isometric contraction of only 10% of the muscle power to maintain tone in the region. Allied to this, a fiber of fibrocartilaginous tissue is emitted in the distal third of the fleshy portion of this muscle and adheres to the epimysium of the extensor carporadialis muscle, transferring the extended configuration to the joints of the carpal region. When this region is extended by around 180°, the accessory ligaments of the digital flexor tendons (superficial and deep) tense them and configure the hyperextended podophalangeal axis, aided by the sesamoid ligament complex and, above all, by the action of the suspensory ligament of the fetlock. This allows the transfer of forces along the limb, keeping it in position during the season with minimal energy expenditure. As a result, equines are able to rest and sleep upright, considering that of the 5 hours of sleep these animals have per day, only between 2 and 3 are REM (*rapid eye movement*), i.e. deep sleep.

CHAPTER 9

ANATOMY AND BIOMECHANICS OF THE APPENDICULAR SKELETON: PELVIC LIMBS

The pelvic limb of horses has well-developed and bulky musculature, responsible for propelling the animal forward, often at great speed (Tabor & Williams, 2018). This segment is anatomically distinct from the ipsilateral limbs up to the line of the hock region, as well as having a system called the reciprocal apparatus, which is very characteristic of the species (Pilliner *et al.*, 2009)

Similarly to the thoracic limbs, the pelvic limbs are divided into two phases in order to better understand the biomechanical and anatomical particularities of each moment (Pilliner *et al.*, 2009). The support phase consists of the limb in contact with the ground and supporting the weight of the horse, while in the suspension phase the limb is suspended in the air, undergoing a forward displacement (protraction). In both moments there are three parts: the cranial phase, the middle phase and the caudal phase, which corresponds to the position of the limb during support or flight (Chateau *et al.*, 2013).

The animal's movement also has a fundamental action of the levers, with the inter-resistant and inter-potent levers acting on the pelvic limb. The second-class levers, such as the trochanteric, patellar and calcaneal levers, generate impulse and absorb impact - but their action depends on the power and stretch of the muscles involved. The third class lever acts specifically during the flight phase by inducing flexion of the limb, but also has actions in the more proximal areas of the limb, which consequently and indirectly also act on the more distal portion of the limb (Denoix, 2014).

This action of the second class lever is only possible due to the reciprocal apparatus, which in horses prevents flexion or extension of the knee without consequent flexion or extension of the hock. Both joints are connected by the tendon of the flexor *digitorum* superficialis muscle and the *peroneus tertius* (fibularis *tertius*) muscle. Because of the action of these two muscles, the movement of the two joints occurs in unison (Tabor & Williams, 2018). In clinical assessments, any injury within the structures of this system will result in significant implications in terms of lameness, such as the rupture of the peroneus tertius, disabling the animal from flexing the hock, while the dislocation of the insertions on the calcaneus of the superficial digital flexor tendon results in a lack of extension of the hock (Denoix, 2014).

During the cranial phase, the impact of the hoof that has just touched the ground is absorbed. Subsequently, an eccentric contraction of various muscle groups, such as the gluteus medius, semitendinosus and semimembranosus, limits the horse's hip flexion. It is important to note that the gluteus medius muscle is the one with the largest volume in the horse, which is an important contributor to propulsion and momentum during locomotion. The knee flexes to a certain extent, with the quadriceps femoris muscle regulating the amplitude of this movement. The hock is stabilized by the superficial digital flexor tendon and the eccentric contraction of the gastrocnemius muscle and other tendinous structures that make up the common calcaneal tendon prevent tarsal collapse.

The intermediate phase is characterized by the stretching of the muscles and the start of the loading phase, storing energy for the following movements. In addition, the joints are limited by various muscle groups, so that there are no injuries or hyperextension of the joints. During propulsion or the caudal phase of support, all the energy stored by the muscles is released and optimized by concentric contraction, which rapidly expands the joint angle. The hip is able to perform a strong extension due to the gluteus medius, followed by knee extension due to the concentric contraction of the quadriceps femoris muscle, which is simultaneous with the extension of the hock with the help of the reciprocal apparatus and the action of the gastrocnemius muscle, together with the caudal femoral muscle group. Thus, the pelvic limb support phase is characterized not only by weight bearing, but also by the participation of all the hip and thigh muscles, which act primarily eccentrically due to stretching during loading and generate concentric contraction (shortening) in propulsion.

During limb suspension, initiated by the caudal phase of flight, the limb retracts to help the joints flex, especially the hip joint, which will suspend the entire limb, through the action of the psoas major and minor muscles, as well as the iliacus muscle (iliopsoas complex) and the muscles cranial to the femur, such as the quadriceps femoris and tensor fascia latae. During the intermediate phase, these muscles will continue to contract concentrically, reducing the joint angle and attenuating hip flexion and, consequently, other distal joints, such as the knee and tarsus, due to the reciprocal apparatus. In addition, the tension caused in the superficial digital flexor muscle triggers flexion of the digital joints, reaching a maximum of simultaneous flexions during the flight phase. Limb protraction ends in the cranial phase, in which the hoof prepares to touch the ground and restart the stride. Mobilization of the hip joint is significantly reduced, while all the other joints rapidly increase their angulations to extend the length of the limb on landing.

CHAPTER 10

ANATOMY AND BIOMECHANICS OF THE AXIAL SKELETON: NECK AND TRUNK

The spine plays a fundamental role in the locomotion of horses, whether they are athletes or not, acting as a suspension bridge between the thoracic and pelvic limbs and supporting the weight of the rider during the execution of riding maneuvers. The spine has a certain flexibility that is indispensable in equestrian sports and has important characteristics in the propulsion phase of the stride (Denoix, 2014). The specific understanding of the biomechanics of the neck, trunk and spine has been the subject of investigation in many texts studying equine movement to try to mitigate the lack of objective knowledge due to the limited range of intrinsic movements at the intervertebral level and the lack of consistency in terminology when discussing the biomechanics or locomotion of the horse. With the advent of more technified methodologies for gait analysis based on the use of wearable sensors, the field of study of these segments has moved from *post-mortem* anatomical dissections to *in vivo* investigations, making it relevant to associate this information with the variety of knowledge about the limbs (Pagger *et al.*, 2010; Schmidburg *et al.*, 2012; Zsoldos *et al.*, 2014).

The neck muscles help to support the thoracic limbs, especially in the pectoral region, due to the absence of a clavicle in horses and the fact that it is the segment with the greatest range of movement along the axial axis of the spine. Basically two muscle groups are involved in suspending the trunk between the thoracic limbs: the serratus muscles, which attach to the upper part of the scapula and support the lower part of the neck (serratus cervical muscle) and the first eight pairs of ribs (serratus thoracis muscle) and the pectoral muscles, which anchor the sternum to the proximal portion of the humerus (ascending pectoral muscle) and the cranial margin of the shoulder (subclavius muscle) (Denoix, 2014). Despite being extensors (*e.g.* splenius) or flexors (*e.g.* brachiocephalic and sternocephalic) of the neck and head, these muscles play an important role in eccentric contraction, since their power and strength are what ensure the lightness of the thoracic limbs during equine locomotion. The efficiency of their concentric contraction ensures the elevation of these segments on take-off before a jump, for example, while the eccentric contraction of these muscles controls the fall of the trunk between the limbs on landing and limits the stresses imposed during the support phase of the stride (Denoix, 2014; Martin *et al.*, 2016).

In the thoracic segment, the extension action is promoted by a large muscle, the erector spinae muscle, which originates caudally in the ilium and extends cranially to the base of the neck, inserting itself in all the vertebrae along its length, as well as in the upper margins of the ribs. The concentric contraction of this muscle results in a powerful extension of the thoracolumbar spine, which brings the spinous processes closer together and, due to its attachment to the wing of the ilium, also results in an upward inclination of the pelvis, inducing extension of the lumbosacral joint (Denoix, 2014; Hobbs *et al.*, 2014). By terminology, epaxial muscles are defined as those located above the vertebral transverse processes and hypaxial muscles are below them.

The lumbosacral joint is of particular importance in spinal mobility, as it is also moved by the powerful action of the gluteus medius muscle, which extends from the lumbar region to the pelvic limb. As previously mentioned, the very action of spinal extension by the epaxial muscles is motivated by the concentric activation of the croup muscles, where the gluteus medius muscle plays a key role in the impulse mechanism of the equine locomotor system, both in different gaits (*e.g. walking,* trotting) and in jumping movements (Zsoldos *et al.*, 2018). In contrast, the flexor musculature of the lumbosacral region includes both the action of the sublumbar muscles (the iliopsoas complex), which promote direct flexion of this joint, as well as the muscles of the abdominal wall, which not only help flex this region, but also thoracolumbar mobility and stabilization of the abdominal wall during stride phases (Robert *et al.*, 2002; Barsanti *et al.*, 2021).

However, movements of the spine are not limited to the longitudinal plane, but also to lateral flexion (lateroflexion) in the horizontal plane, which is almost always associated with secondary rotation. This mobility is not induced by specific muscles, but by the action of flexors and extensors, as mentioned above, when they promote asymmetrical concentric contraction on one side of the spine, resulting in flexion of the spine to the same side (Denoix, 2014). Along the axial axis, the cervical region also has the greatest mobility in this type of angular action (Zsoldos *et al.*, 2010). Lateral flexion in the thoracolumbar region is most pronounced in the caudal half of the thoracic region, which is the result of unilateral contraction of the erector spinae muscle and the oblique abdominal muscles (Faber *et al.*, 2000). In the lumbosacral joint, lateroflexion is practically non-existent (Audigié *et al.*, 1999).

The spine, however, does not bend, but performs torsional movements in the transverse plane. This angular action that occurs around the vertebral axis is often associated with lateroflexion movements and is defined by the side to which the ventral aspect of the vertebrae moves in relation to the pelvis and hind limbs, which are fixed structures during the animal's support on the ground (Zaneb, 2013). These movements can be active, initiated by concentric muscle contraction, or they can also be a passive reaction to the positioning of the limbs where, in this case, eccentric contraction of the rotating muscles controls the amount of movement (Denoix, 2014). In the thoracolumbar spine, the area that performs the most rotation is the caudal half of the thoracic region, with the oblique abdominal muscles being the most active in these movements, whereas in the lumbosacral region, rotation is significantly limited due to the vertebrae being blocked by ligaments during flexion and extension (Mackechnie-Guire & Pfau, 2021).

REFERENCES BIBLIOGRAPHIC

ADELMAN, M.; THOMPSON, K. **Introduction to equestrian cultures in global and local contexts.** In Equestrian Cultures in Global and Local Contexts (pp. 1-14). Springer, Cham. 2017.

ALLUM, J. H.; ADKIN, A. L. **Improvements in trunk sway observed for stance and gait tasks during recovery from an acute unilateral peripheral vestibular deficit.** Audiology and Neurotology, 8(5), 286-302. 2003.

ALSIRI, N.; CRAMP, M., BARNETT, S.; PALMER, S. **Gait biomechanics in joint hypermobility syndrome: a spatiotemporal, kinematic and kinetic analysis.** Musculoskeletal Care, 18(3), 301-314. 2020.

AMADIO, A. C.; DUARTE, M. **Fundamentos biomecânicos para a análise do movimento humano.** São Paulo: Biomechanics Laboratory/EEFUSP, 10. 1996.

ANTONIOLI, M. L. **Effect of hoof trimming on hoof biometry and thoracic joint angles of Mangalarga females.** 2019.

AUDIGIÉ, F.; POURCELOT, P.; DEGUEURCE, C.; DENOIX, J. M.; GEIGER, D. **Kinematics of the equine back: flexion-extension movements in sound trotting horses.** Equine Veterinary Journal, 31(S30), 210-213. 1999.

BACK, W.; SCHAMHARDT, H. C.; SAVELBERG, H. H. C. M.; VAN DEN BOGERT, A. J.; BRUIN, G.; HARTMAN, W.; BARNEVELD, A. **How the horse moves: 1. Significance of graphical representations of equine forelimb kinematics.** Equine Veterinary Journal, 27(1), 31-38. 1995.

BAKER, R. **Gait analysis methods in rehabilitation.** Journal of neuroengineering and rehabilitation, 3(1), 1-10. 2006.

BARREY, E. **Methods, applications and limitations of gait analysis in horses.** The veterinary journal, 157(1), 7-22. 1999.

BARSANTI, R. R.; FONSECA, B. P. A.; SILVATTI, A. P.; SIMONATO, S. P.; PEREIRA, V. G.; MARTINS, N. A.; VIEIRA, E. G. **Descriptive electromyography signals analysis of equine longissimus dorsi, rectus abdominis and gluteus medius muscles during maneuvers used to activate the core.** Arquivo Brasileiro de Medicina Veterinária e Zootecnia, 73, 843-852. 2021.

SHERBURN, M.; BØ, K. **Evaluation of female pelvic-floor muscle function and strength.** Pherhys T, 85(3), 269-282. 2005.

BRETAS, M. S.; BERGMANN, J.A.G.; PROCÓPIO, A.M. **Description of anatomical points for taking linear and angular measurements in Mangalarga Marchador horses.** In: Scientific Initiation Week, 2003, Belo Horizonte. Proceedings. Belo Horizonte: UFMG. Cd Rom. 2003.

CASADEI, K.; KIEL, J. **Anthropometric measurement.** StatPearls [Internet]. 2020.

CASTELLI, A.; PAOLINI, G.; CEREATTI, A.; DELLA CROCE, U. **A 2D markerless gait analysis methodology: validation on healthy subjects.** Computational and mathematical methods in medicine. 2015.

CESERACCIU, E.; SAWACHA, Z.; COBELLI, C. **Comparison of markerless and marker-based motion capture technologies through simultaneous data collection during gait: proof of concept.** PloS one, 9(3), e87640. 2014.

CHATEAU, H.; ROBIN, D.; SIMONELLI, T.; PACQUET, L.; POURCELOT, P.; FALALA, S.; CREVIER-DENOIX, N. **Design and validation of a dynamometric horseshoe for the measurement of three-dimensional ground reaction force on a moving horse.** Journal of biomechanics, 42(3), 336-340. 2009.

CHATEAU, H.; CAMUS, M.; HOLDEN-DOUILLY, L.; FALALA, S.; RAVARY, B., VERGARI, C.; CREVIER-DENOIX, N. **Kinetics of the forelimb in horses** circling on different ground surfaces at the trot. The Veterinary Journal, 198, e20-e26. 2013.

CHUNG, P. Y. M.; NG, G. Y. F. Comparison between an accelerometer and a three-dimensional motion analysis system for the detection of movement. Physiotherapy, 98(3), 256-259. 2012.

CLAYTON, H.; SCHAMHARDT, H.C. Measurement techniques for gait analysis. In: Back, W.; Clayton, H. Equine locomotion. London, W.B. Saunders. p.55-75. 2001.

CLAYTON, H. M.; SHA, D.; STICK, J.; ELVIN, N. 3D kinematics of the equine metacarpophalangeal joint at walk and trot. Veterinary and Comparative Orthopaedics and Traumatology, 2(02), 86-91. 2007.

CLAYTON, H. M. Horse species symposium: Biomechanics of the exercising horse. Journal of animal science, 94(10), 4076-4086. 2016.

CLAYTON, H. M.; HOBBS, S. J. The role of biomechanical analysis of horse and rider in equitation science. Applied Animal Behavior Science, 190, 123-132. 2017.

CLAYTON, H. M.; HOBBS, S. J. Ground reaction forces: The sine qua non of legged locomotion. Journal of equine veterinary science, 76, 25-35. 2019.

CRUZ, A. M.; MANINCHEDDA, U. E.; BURGER, D.; WANDA, S.; VIDONDO, B. Repeatability of gait pattern variables measured by use of extremity-mounted inertial measurement units in nonlame horses during trotting. American journal of veterinary research, 78(9), 1011-1018. 2017.

DAKIN, S. G., JESPERS, K., WARNER, S., O'HARA, L. K., DUDHIA, J., GOODSHIP, A. E., ... & SMITH, R. K. W. The relationship between in vivo limb and in vitro tendon mechanics after injury: a potential novel clinical tool for monitoring tendon repair. Equine veterinary journal, 43(4), 418-423. 2011.

DAUBE, J. R.; RUBIN, D. I. **Needle electromyography.** Muscle & Nerve: Official Journal of the American Association of Electrodiagnostic Medicine, 39(2), 244-270. 2009.

DE GODOI, F. N.; DE ALMEIDA, F. Q.; TORAL, F. L. B.; DE MIRANDA, A. L. S.; KAIPPER, R. R.; BERGMANN, J. A. G. **Repeatability of kinematics traits of free jumping in Brazilian sport horses.** Livestock Science, 168, 1-8. 2014.

DE LUCA, C. **Electromyography.** Encyclopedia of medical devices and instrumentation. 2006.

DE LUCA, C. J.; GILMORE, L. D.; KUZNETSOV, M.; ROY, S. H. **Filtering the surface EMG signal: Movement artifact and baseline noise contamination.** Journal of biomechanics, 43(8), 1573-1579. 2010.

DENOIX, J. M. **Biomechanics and physical training of the horse.** CRC Press. 2014.

DYSON, S.; ELLIS, A. D.; MACKECHNIE-GUIRE, R.; DOUGLAS, J.; BONDI, A.; HARRIS, P. **The influence of rider: horse bodyweight ratio and rider-horse-saddle fit on equine gait and behavior: A pilot study.** Equine Veterinary Education, 32(10), 527-539. 2020.

FONSECA, M. G. **Mangalarga Marchador: morphometric, kinematic and genetic study of the beaten gait and paced gait.** 2018.

EGAN, S.; BRAMA, P.; MCGRATH, D. **Research trends in equine movement analysis, future opportunities and potential barriers in the digital age: A scoping review from 1978 to 2018.** Equine Veterinary Journal, 51(6), 813-824. 2019.

FABER, M.; SCHAMHARDT, H.; VAN WEEREN, R.; JOHNSTON, C.; ROEPSTORFF, L.; BARNEVELD, A. B. **Basic three-dimensional kinematics of

the vertebral column of horses walking on a treadmill. American journal of veterinary research, 61(4), 399-406. 2000.

FAULKNER, J. A. **Terminology for contractions of muscles during shortening, while isometric, and during lengthening.** Journal of Applied Physiology, 95(2), 455-459. 2003.

GOUBEL, F. **Muscular compliance during isometric contraction.** Journal de Physiologie, 74(6), 609-614. 1978.

GRAZIANO, A. **Biomecânica: fundamentos e aplicações na Educação Física Escolar.** EDUCA, UP. 2008.

GRIFFIN, T. M.; KRAM, R.; WICKLER, S. J.; HOYT, D. F. **Biomechanical and energetic determinants of the walk-trot transition in horses.** Journal of Experimental Biology, 207(24), 4215-4223. 2004.

GUSTÅS, P.; JOHNSTON, C.; ROEPSTORFF, L.; DREVEMO, S.; LANSHAMMAR, H. **Relationships between fore-and hindlimb ground reaction force and hoof deceleration patterns in trotting horses.** Equine veterinary journal, 36(8), 737-742. 2004.

HATZE, H. **The meaning of the term" biomechanics".** Journal of biomechanics, 7(2), 189-190. 1974.

HENLEY, W. E.; ROGERS, K.; HARKINS, L.; WOOD, J. L. N. **A comparison of survival models for assessing risk of racehorse fatality.** Preventive Veterinary Medicine, 74(1), 3-20. 2006.

HILDEBRAND, M. **Analysis of asymmetrical gaits.** Journal of Mammalogy, 58(2), 131-156. 1997.

HOBBS, S. J.; CLAYTON, H. M. **Sagittal plane ground reaction forces, center of pressure and center of mass in trotting horses.** The Veterinary Journal, 198, e14-e19. 2013.

HOBBS, S. J.; RICHARDS, J.; CLAYTON, H. M. **The effect of center of mass location on sagittal plane moments around the center of mass in trotting horses.** Journal of Biomechanics, 47(6), 1278-1286. 2014.

HUG, F. **Can muscle coordination be precisely studied by surface electromyography?** Journal of electromyography and kinesiology, 21(1), 1-12. 2011.

HUSSNI, C. A.; WISSDORF, H.; NICOLETT, J. L. D. M. **Gait variations in Mangalarga Marchador horses.** Ciência Rural, 26, 91-95. 1996.

JOHNSON, J. L.; MOORE-COLYER, M. **The relationship between range of motion of lumbosacral flexion-extension and canter velocity of horses on a treadmill.** Equine veterinary journal, 41(3), 301-303. 2009.

KAMEN, G.; GABRIEL, D. A. **Essentials of electromyography.** Human Kinetics Publishers. 2009.

KILBOURNE, B. M.; HOFFMAN, L. C. **Scale effects between body size and limb design in quadrupedal mammals.** PloS one, 8(11), e78392. 2013.

LEACH, D. H., & DAGG, A. I. **Evolution of equine locomotion research.** Equine Veterinary Journal, 15(2), 87-92. 1983.

LILEY, H.; ZHANG, J.; FIRTH, E.; FERNANDEZ, J.; BESIER, T. **Using partial least squares regression as a predictive tool in describing equine third metacarpal bone shape.** Computer methods in BiomeChaniCs and BiomediCal engineering, 20(15), 1609-1612. 2017.

LU, T. W.; CHANG, C. F. **Biomechanics of human movement and its clinical applications.** The Kaohsiung journal of medical sciences, 28, S13-S25. 2012.

MACKECHNIE-GUIRE, R.; PFAU, T. **Differential rotational movement and symmetry values of the thoracolumbosacral region in high-level dressage horses when trotting.** Plos one, 16(5), e0251144. 2021.

MAREY, E. J. **Animal mechanism: a treatise on terrestrial and aerial locomotion** (Vol. 11). Henry S. King & Company. 1874.

MARTIN, P.; CHEZE, L.; POURCELOT, P.; DESQUILBET, L.; DURAY, L.; CHATEAU, H. **Effect of the rider position during rising trot on the horse's biomechanics (back and trunk kinematics and pressure under the saddle).** Journal of biomechanics, 49(7), 1027-1033. 2016.

MCHENRY, M. J.; HEDRICK, T. L. **The science and technology of kinematic measurements in a century of Journal of Experimental Biology.** Journal of Experimental Biology, 226(Suppl_1), jeb245147. 2023.

MEERSHOEK, L. S., SCHAMHARDT, H. C., ROEPSTORFF, L., & JOHNSTON, C. **Forelimb tendon loading during jump landings and the influence of fence height.** Equine Veterinary Journal, 33(S33), 6-10. 2001.

MICHELINI, A.; ESHRAGHI, A.; ANDRYSEK, J. **Two-dimensional video gait analysis: A systematic review of reliability, validity, and best practice considerations.** Prosthetics and Orthotics International, 44(4), 245-262. 2020.

MILLS, K. R. **The basics of electromyography.** Journal of Neurology, Neurosurgery & Psychiatry, 76(suppl 2), ii32-ii35. 2005.

MIRÓ, F.; VIVO, J.; CANO, R.; DIZ, A.; GALISTEO, A. M. **Walk and trot in the horse at driving: kinematic adaptation of its natural gaits.** Animal Research, 55(6), 603-613. 2006.

MUNOZ-NATES, F.; CHATEAU, H.; VAN HAMME, A.; CAMUS, M.; PAUCHARD, M.; RAVARY-PLUMIOEN, B.; CREVIER-DENOIX, N. **Accelerometric and dynamometric measurements of the impact shock of the equine forelimb and hindlimb at high-speed trot on six different tracks-Preliminary study in one horse.** Computer Methods in Biomechanics and Biomedical Engineering, 18(Suppl. 1), 2012-2013. 2015.

MURRAY, R.; GUIRE, R.; FISHER, M.; FAIRFAX, V. **A bridle designed to avoid peak pressure locations under the headpiece and noseband is associated with more uniform pressure and increased carpal and tarsal flexion, compared with the horse's usual bridle.** Journal of Equine Veterinary Science, 35(11-12), 947-955. 2015.

MUYBRIDGE, E. **Animals in Motion.** Dover, New York (with reprints from the 1899 original). 1957.

NOCERA, I.; SGORBINI, M.; GRACIA-CALVO, L. A.; CACINI, M.; VITALE, V.; CITI, S. **A novel dynamometer for the standardization of the force applied during distal forelimb flexion tests in horses.** Equine Veterinary Education, 33(9), 484-488. 2021.

OLSEN, E.; PFAU, T.; RITZ, C. **Functional limits of agreement applied as a novel method comparison tool for accuracy and precision of inertial measurement unit derived displacement of the distal limb in horses.** Journal of Biomechanics, 46(13), 2320-2325. 2013.

OTT, J. **Iron horses: Leland Stanford, Eadweard Muybridge, and the industrialized eye.** Oxford Art Journal, 28(3), 407-428. 2005.

PADULO, J., LAFFAYE, G., ARDIGÒ, L. P., & CHAMARI, K. **Concentric and eccentric: muscle contraction or exercise?** Journal of human kinetics, 37(1), 5-6. 2013.

PAGGER, H.; SCHMIDBURG, I.; PEHAM, C.; LICKA, T. **Determination of the stiffness of the equine cervical spine.** The Veterinary Journal, 186(3), 338-341. 2010.

PARK, S. H.; CHOI, S. J.; LEE, K. S.; PARK, H. Y. **Waist circumference and waist-to-height ratio as predictors of cardiovascular disease risk in Korean adults.** Circulation Journal, 73(9), 1643-1650. 2009.

PATAY-HORVÁTH, A. **Greek Geometric Animal Figurines and the Origins of the Ancient Olympic Games.** In Arts (Vol. 9, No. 1, p. 20). Multidisciplinary Digital Publishing Institute. 2020.

PAYNE, R. C.; VEENMAN, P.; WILSON, A. M. **The role of the extrinsic thoracic limb muscles in equine locomotion.** Journal of Anatomy, 206(2), 193-204. 2005.

PAZ, C. F. R.; FERNANDES, T. L. B.; PAOLUCCI, L. A.; DE OLIVEIRA, A. D. P. L.; MARÓSTICA, T. P.; DE LIMA, M. P. A.; FALEIROS, R. R. **Stride kinematic changes in laminitic horses treated with three different types of hoof orthopedic devices.** Semina: Ciências Agrárias, 40(6Supl3), 3755-3762. 2019.

PEREIRA, J. P. D. C. **Kinematic Analysis of Horses on Two Different Surfaces With and Without Rider Influence**. Doctoral dissertation, University of Lisbon, Portugal. 2019.

PFAU, T. **Sensor-based equine gait analysis: more than meets the eye?** UK-Vet Equine, 3(3), 102-112. 2019.

PILLINER, S.; ELMHURST, S.; DAVIES, Z. **The horse in motion: the anatomy and physiology of equine locomotion.** John Wiley & Sons. 2009.

PRATT, G. W.; O'CONNOR Jr, J. T. **Force plate studies of equine biomechanics.** American Journal of Veterinary Research, 37(11), 1251-1255. 1976.

RAMACHANDRAN, M.; LEE, P. **Basic concepts in biomechanics.** In Basic orthopaedic sciences (pp. 233-244). CRC Press. 2018.

RASH, G. S.; QUESADA, P. **Electromyography fundamentals.** Retrieved February, 4. 2003.

ROBERT, C.; VALETTE, J.P.; POURCELOT, P.; AUDIGIE, F.; DENOIX, J.M. **Effects of trotting speed on muscle activity and kinematics in saddlehorses.** Equine Vet J. S34:295-301. 2002.

ROBILLIARD, J. J.; PFAU, T.; WILSON, A. M. **Gait characterization and classification in horses.** Journal of Experimental Biology, 210(2), 187-197. 2007.

ROBIN, D.; CHATEAU, H.; PACQUET, L.; FALALA, S.; VALETTE, J. P.; POURCELOT, P.; CREVIER-DENOIX, N. **Use of a 3D dynamometric horseshoe to assess the effects of an all-weather waxed track and a crushed sand track at high-speed trot: preliminary study.** Equine Veterinary Journal, 41(3), 253-256. 2009.

ROEPSTORFF, L.; WIESTNER, T.; WEISHAUPT, M. A.; EGENVALL, E. **Comparison of microgyro-based measurements of equine metatarsal/metacarpal bone to a high-speed video locomotion analysis system during treadmill locomotion.** The Veterinary Journal, 198, e157-e160. 2013.

SANDAU, M.; KOBLAUCH, H.; MOESLUND, T. B.; AANÆS, H.; ALKJÆR, T.; SIMONSEN, E. B. **Markerless motion capture can provide reliable 3D gait kinematics in the sagittal and frontal plane.** Medical engineering & physics, 36(9), 1168-1175. 2014.

SANTOS, L. U. D. **Biomechanical analysis of gait in mangalarga marchador foals in the first 15 days of life.** 2018.

SAPONE, M.; MARTIN, P.; BEN MANSOUR, K.; CHATEAU, H.; MARIN, F. **The protraction and retraction angles of horse limbs: an estimation during trotting using inertial sensors.** Sensors, 21(11), 3792. 2021.

SCHMIDBURG, I.; PAGGER, H.; ZSOLDOS, R. R.; MEHNEN, J.; PEHAM, C.; LICKA, T. F. **Movement associated reduction of spatial capacity of the equine cervical vertebral canal.** The Veterinary Journal, 192(3), 525-528. 2012.

SIMONATO, S. P.; BERNARDINA, G. R.; FERREIRA, L. C.; SILVATTI, A. P.; BARCELOS, K. M.; DA FONSECA, B. P. **3D kinematic of the thoracolumbar spine in Mangalarga Marchador horses performing the marcha batida gait and being led by hand-A preliminary report.** Plos one, 16(7), e0253697. 2021.

SMITH, K. **Here's how to smooth the transitions from four beats to two, two beats to three, from slow motion to speed.** Equus Magazine, v.230, p.27-32. 1996.

SOARES, C. D. M. **Biomechanical analysis of the gait of mangalarga marchador foals at 30 and 180 days of age.** 2017.

TABOR, G.; WILLIAMS, J. **Equine rehabilitation: a review of trunk and hind limb muscle activity and exercise selection.** Journal of Equine Veterinary Science, 60, 97-103. 2018.

THOMAS, D.; AYSYLU, G.; NICOLE, A.; GOTTFRIED, B.; WALTER, K. **The use of image data in the assessment of equine conformation-limitations and solutions.** Visual observation and analysis of Vertebrate and Insect Behavior. Springer. 2014.

TORRES-PÉREZ, Y.; GÓMEZ-PACHÓN, E. Y.; CUENCA-JIMÉNEZ, F. **Horse's gait motion analysis system based on videometry.** Ciencia y Agricultura, 13(2), 83-94. 2016.

UGBOLUE, U. C.; PAPI, E.; KALIARNTAS, K. T.; KERR, A.; EARL, L.; POMEROY, V. M.; ROWE, P. J. **The evaluation of an inexpensive, 2D, video-based gait assessment system for clinical use.** Gait & posture, 38(3), 483-489. 2013.

ULIJASZEK, S. J.; KERR, D. A. **Anthropometric measurement error and the assessment of nutritional status.** British Journal of Nutrition, 82(3), 165-177. 1999.

USPENSKII, V. D. **Anatomical-Physiological Analysis of Limb in Allure and Its Practical Significance**, Tr. Statovsk Zoovet. Inst, 4, 109-115. 1953.

VAN WEEREN, P. R., BRAMA, P. A., & BARNEVELD, A. **Exercise at young age may influence the final quality of the equine musculoskeletal system.** In Proceedings (Vol. 46, pp. 29-35). 2000.

VAN WEEREN, R. **Equine biomechanics: From an adjunct of art to a science in its own right.** Equine Veterinary Journal, 44(5), 506-508. 2012.

VON PEINEN, K.; WIESTNER, T.; BOGISCH, S.; ROEPSTORFF, L.; VAN WEEREN, P. R.; WEISHAUPT, M. A. **Relationship between the forces acting on the horse's back and the movements of rider and horse while walking on a treadmill.** Equine Veterinary Journal, 41(3), 285-291. 2009.

WHITTLE, M. W. **Clinical gait analysis: A review.** Human movement science, 15(3), 369-387. 1996.

WIJNBERG, I. D.; FRANSSEN, H. **The potential and limitations of quantitative electromyography in equine medicine.** The Veterinary Journal, 209, 23-31. 2016.

WILLIAMS, J. M. **Electromyography in the horse: A useful technology?** Journal of Equine Veterinary Science, 60, 43-58. 2018.

ZANEB, H.; PEHAM, C.; STANEK, C. **Functional anatomy and biomechanics of the equine thoracolumbar spine: a review.** Turkish Journal of Veterinary and Animal Sciences, 37(4), 380-389. 2013.

ZSOLDOS, R. R.; GROESEL, M.; KOTSCHWAR, A.; KOTSCHWAR, A. B.; LICKA, T.; PEHAM, C. **A preliminary modelling study on the equine cervical spine with inverse kinematics at walk.** Equine Veterinary Journal, 42, 516-522. 2010.

ZSOLDOS, R. R.; KRÜGER, B.; LICKA, T. F. **From maturity to old age: tasks of daily life require a different muscle use in horses.** Comparative exercise physiology, 10(2), 75-88. 2014.

ZSOLDOS, R. R.; VOEGELE, A.; KRUEGER, B.; SCHROEDER, U.; WEBER, A.; LICKA, T. F. **Long term consistency and location specificity of equine gluteus medius muscle activity during locomotion on the treadmill.** BMC veterinary research, 14(1), 1-10. 2018.

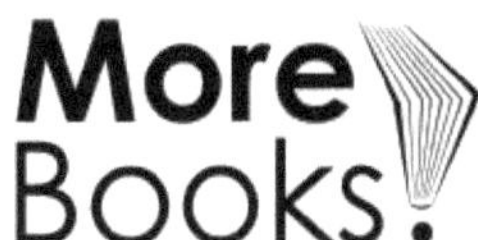

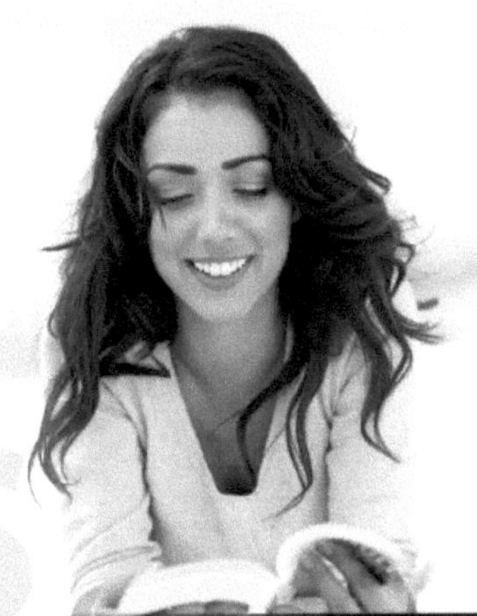

I want morebooks!

Buy your books fast and straightforward online - at one of world's fastest growing online book stores! Environmentally sound due to Print-on-Demand technologies.

Buy your books online at
www.morebooks.shop

Kaufen Sie Ihre Bücher schnell und unkompliziert online – auf einer der am schnellsten wachsenden Buchhandelsplattformen weltweit! Dank Print-On-Demand umwelt- und ressourcenschonend produzi ert.

Bücher schneller online kaufen
www.morebooks.shop

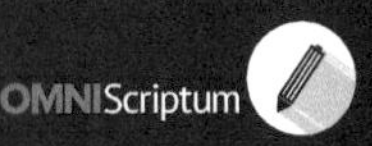

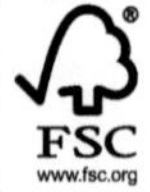

Printed by Books on Demand GmbH, Norderstedt / Germany